My Daughter
Died Laughing

A memoir about Ashley Long's life and a book about awareness of the dangers of inhaling helium

My Daughter Died Laughing

Ashley Long's story

LORI EARP

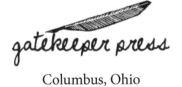

Columbus, Ohio

My Daughter Died Laughing: Ashley Long's Story

Published by Gatekeeper Press
3971 Hoover Rd. Suite 77
Columbus, OH 43123-2839
www.GatekeeperPress.com

ISBN: 9781619846968
eISBN: 9781619846975

Printed in the United States of America

Contents

Ashley Jean Long

I WAS 21 WHEN Ashley was born and I never wanted anything more in my life. I was completely prepared to bring her into the world. We couldn't wait to meet her. She would be the first granddaughter born on both sides of our family. Sometimes when I think about her, I want to remember her directly, as if I could still talk to her. At those times, I find myself talking to her as if she were still here.

From the beginning, Ashley, you took your sweet time getting here though. Two weeks after my due date and you still weren't here. So the doctor had to start inducing labor. There was nothing quick about that. The next 25 hours would be the longest, most painful time in my life. All of the women in our family were there that day. Even your grandpas and Uncles awaited your arrival.

Ashley Jean Long was born at Rogue Valley hospital in Medford, Oregon on January 9th 1998. She weighed 7lbs 11oz. She was a jaundiced baby so she needed to be in the Wallaby for the first couple of weeks. We were able to rent one when we brought her home. Jaundice just meant your color was a little off and you needed a certain light to fix it.

You were perfect, though. You had all your fingers and toes. When you were born, you had brown hair and brown eyes. Your blonde hair quickly came in full of curls.

From the moment Ashley was born, my life changed. My heart was filled with so much love for her. When you love someone you put their needs ahead of your own. She was unconditionally loved from the moment she was born. She was a happy and content baby. She slept through the night and was rarely sick. I had her nursery decorated with the artist Anne Geddes' babies who were dressed up like flowers or butterflies. It was adorable. Ashley took her first steps at around 10 months.

On her first birthday, we invited all the family to get together at her Grandma Connie's house. She was so excited to have all the attention on her. Tore into her presents and when it came time for the cake she became dainty—she didn't want to get messy. We had a special mini cake made just for her. She cried when the cake got all over her, but she still loved eating it.

When Ashley was a toddler she had a special quilt blanket that her grandma Debbie had made for her. She never went anywhere without it. She would rub the corner on her lips when she was restless or trying to fall asleep. Ashley was a happy and content child, with beautiful blonde curls, squeezable cheeks and big brown eyes. She was always a joy to have. Full of curiosity and eager to learn, she always captured the attention in the room. She loved to gather everyone together when she was two and she would stand on her little chair and sing "Happy Birthday!" along with "The Itsy Bitsy Spider!" She loved playing dress up or "cooking" in her little kitchen. She was so silly and entertaining and all of us adored her. She was so full of life.

When she was 1 years old I took her to the amusement park, Great America, with her Grandma Connie and Aunt Brandi. It was the 4th of July. We watched the fireworks from the middle of rides. I took you to Hollywood when you were 2 and we went to Universal Studios. Ashley and I took a picture together under the giant Hard Rock café guitar. We also took a picture together under the Hollywood sign.

When Ashley was 3-and-a-half, her father and I split up. Her father moved up to Washington shortly after. When he moved, she was unable to see him for quite a while. He never made it down to visit and we never went there. They wrote a few letters back and forth. She was able to talk with him on the phone when he called. She lived with me from then on in Grants Pass. The majority of her family lived there from either side of the family. I always stayed close with her relatives on her father's side. I wanted them to know who she was and to be able to watch her grow up. I always felt it was important for kids to grow up close to their family.

Just before Ashley turned 4 years old I met her step-dad, Justin. At first she was curious and a little shy. Soon after, they both found they had a special place in each other's hearts. Justin had an 8-year-old son named T.J. and Ashley was so excited at the possibility of having a brother. The four of us soon became a family. She loved going to Justin's softball games with me. She'd get her words mixed up and when he'd make a home run she'd yell, "TOUCHDOWN!" It was so adorable.

Ashley learned how to ride a bicycle when she was about 6 years old. Justin taught her to ride without the training wheels. She loved that now she could go fast. Around this time, her Grandma Laura began teaching her how to swim. Our neighbor had a pool and Ashley loved swimming with her.

When it was time for kindergarten Ashley panicked. The first day of school scared her to death. She didn't want me to leave her side. It took a couple of weeks before I could walk her to the classroom and say "goodbye" without her crying. She was shy and seemingly attached at my hip. We were always very close and spent about every day together. This made it hard when it came time for school. She didn't know how to be without me and it was scary for her to be suddenly with a group of kids. She had a hard time approaching them to ask if they wanted to play.

In time she managed to break out of her shell and always made friends. I think she picked up her habit of rubbing her mouth with her shirt when she was adjusting to being separated during school hours. I think she found comfort in doing this; it helped to calm her. She had that habit her entire life. When she was younger, she was very gullible and believed everything she was told. We used to tease her and tell her the factory smoke going into the sky was how clouds were made. Or that it was raining in front of us only, and then he'd turn on the wiper blades and the car mister. She had quite an imagination. When we drove along the freeway, Justin liked to run the tires along the safety line. The grooved edge on the road makes a loud sound when you drive on it. Justin liked to tease Ashley and tell her the sound was a dinosaur farting. She'd get all serious and quiet listening for more.

Mariah was born when Ashley was 5. Ashley couldn't wait to be a big sister. She was always my best helper. Always wanting to hold Mariah every chance she got. She loved helping her learn to crawl and walk. She took great pride in being a big sister. Mariah was the only sibling she lived with so naturally they were the closest. They were always together—Mariah was her shadow. Ashley was the best big sissy, always looking out for her sister, making sure she was ok. She taught her sister Mariah so much.

They loved to dress up and take pictures together. They were always making videos up and recording each other. Ashley loved singing with Mariah. They could sing and dance for hours. They spent a lot of time designing fashion outfits and making up different styles. Ashley was always fixing Mariah's hair and Mariah wanted only Ashley's opinion on how she looked for the day.

Ashley's father's side of the family lived up in Washington. Her father remarried and soon she had more sisters. She would visit them a couple of times a year. When Ashley was around the age of 10 her dad taught her to catch her first fish. She was proud of that moment. The Transformer's movie was one of Ashley's favorite movies that her dad took her to see. She liked to save the ticket stubs as souvenirs. She liked cooking with her stepmother, Alisa, and helping out with her little sisters when she'd visit. Alisa introduced her to many different kinds of foods that Ashley enjoyed. Of course her sisters all adored her. She would spend her time up there in Washington playing with them and making them laugh. They were all very young, just toddlers when Ashley was alive. Fortunately, she took many pictures of them. When they are older they will cherish them and will see how much she loved them. She was a proud sister and grateful to have them. Ashley had so much love for all her family.

When Ashley was 7 years old, Justin and I got married. She was our little bright and shining flower girl. Our theme colors were purple, silver and white. She wore a purple flowered head-piece in her hair and carried a white silk basket filled with purple petals. She danced her tail off with her siblings and cousins that night. She loved Justin and T. J. and couldn't wait to be a family with them. Our home was filled with nothing but love and happiness. We were a family.

T.J., her step-brother, was able to visit us each month so they grew very close. They loved to sit together. He'd play his guitar and she would make up songs. I remember when he visited they had this game they'd play. He would change her password on her I-pod and sometimes it would take hours for her to figure it out. There was lots of teasing, and joking around. She bragged about her step-brother to all her friends. She looked up to him so much. Her friends thought he was so cute and would crush on him. Of course, siblings argue and fight but overall they loved each other.

As a family we tried to spend as much time together making as many memories as possible. We were always at the river or a lake during summers, swimming and barbequing. We took pictures and made memories.

Your grandparents have always been a big part of your life. You and your grandma, Debbie, were always gardening when you visited her. Your grandpa, Tom, would take you to the movies. You also loved going out on the lake with your grandpa Tom. Sometimes your cousin, Kaleb, who was a year younger, would come. He let you steer the boat. You thought you were so cool. Your grandma, Connie, liked to take you on the First Friday's of the month celebration. In Grants Pass, they have First Friday and all the stores downtown stay open late. They have art exhibits and lots of food and drinks.

Ashley also loved to paint with her Grandma Connie. She loved it when Grandpa Rick would show her all his crystals and the cool rocks he'd find rock hunting. She loved all the stories he had to tell. She loved going out to their property with the family. Swimming in the creek behind their house and bonfires at night were good times. She has many cousins and lots of aunts and uncles living in the valley, along with Grandmas and Grandpas, all full of love.

Ashley held a special place in her heart for her Aunt Bobbi and Cousin Vanessa. They would take her with them to church and afterwards they would have lunch at The Olive Garden. This was another favorite restaurant of hers. "Nessie" as Ashley called her, and Ashley would stay up all night, laughing, singing songs and making videos of each other, just being as silly as possible. Ashley looked up to Nessie—she was her favorite cousin. They made so many memories together, being complete nerds. Ashley's Aunt Michelle was the one she looked most like. Ashley adored her, loved spending time with her. They looked so much alike that strangers would think she was Michelle's daughter. Michelle always did Ashley's hair in different styles. They had always been very close her whole life.

Ashley was able to be close with most of her cousins and family. She was close her entire life with her cousins, Jeremiah, Zach and Erin. These are my brother Rick and my sister Brandi's kids. We had all been raising our families in the Rogue Valley their whole lives. We kept our kids close, always hanging out together. We gathered together for the holidays. Halloween, Christmas, and Easter were favorites. There are a few hundred people directly related to Ashley living in the valley we live in. With so much family around growing up, Ashley always had something fun to attend. She loved being able to spend time with family—it was her favorite thing to do.

Over the years, due to the economy, we moved back and forth a few times, between the town of Medford and my home town of Grants Pass. They are about 30 min apart, but Ashley had to meet new friends every few years. I always felt bad for her, but she was tough and brave and would always make friends. She was a social butterfly. She got along with everybody.

School came easy for Ashley. She was like sponge. Everything that she was taught she remembered. She never had any problems doing her homework. Which was a good thing because I'm horrible with math and would have been no help. Her teachers always had good comments and kind words to say. She had excellent grades throughout school, averaging A's and B's. She would go above and beyond with extra credit to get the grade. Her favorite teacher was Mrs. Roe from 2nd grade. Mrs. Roe was from Highland Elementary School in Grants Pass. Ashley's best talents were art and writing. She was very creative. Math seemed to come easy to her, too. There wasn't a subject she disliked.

In middle school she took an interest in photography. She was always taking pictures. She knew how to capture the beauty in anything. She could focus in on a single leaf with dew drops on it, making it look like something from a National Geographic magazine. She also loved fashion. She and I would watch the designing shows and she was always sketching different ideas. She had a love for art, drawing, and poetry. She was very expressive in anything she did. Her personality always showed through her art.

She had a big interest in eyes. She was always drawing different types. Her cartoon eyes always had a double pupil in them. This was like her trademark—she loved it. There was a picture of an eye close up in black and white she made with Mariah and her head's in the middle. Around the edge of the eye, she put the words, "Just open your eyes and see the world is beautiful." She was very creative. I love everything she made. I've saved everything she made all through school and I'm so grateful to have them now. Seeing your child through their art really lets you know who they are and how they are feeling inside. By Ashley's art, we could clearly tell she was a happy girl and completely loved. Her art was always full of color and detail. She took great pride in her drawings.

She also had a big love for animals. She had pets from cats to dogs and her favorite was our dog Sadie. She took her out on walks as much as she could and loved grooming her.

Also in Middle school Ashley started being more self-conscious about what others thought. Always taking extra time in the mirror making sure her look was ok. On the way to school, she would flip the visor down in the truck to look in the mirror one more time. She became aware of name brands and what other kids were wearing to school. Every teen goes through it, the pressure of fitting in. It is especially difficult being the new girl in school, when all eyes seem to be on you. I think because of her experiencing this a few times, she held a soft spot in her heart for the next new kid. When it came to loyalty and friendship Ashley was always there for her friends. She always made others feel equal and accepted. She would stand up for the underdog getting picked on. She believed everyone's life mattered. She did not agree with bullying!

Ashley's poem from her 8th grade yearbook

Your Life Matters to me
Just like any other day
Life may take you down sometimes but,
You will always have me by your side
To bring you back up
Wipe away your tears and tell you
You're stronger than you think you are.
My life would never be the same
Without you around.
I just want you to see
Your life matters to me . . .

By, Ashley Jean Long

Ashley had excellent grades all through school. By the 8th grade, she had a 3.5 GPA and was a member of the honor roll and a Top Cat in her school. We were very proud of her. Things hadn't been easy. She managed to stay focused through it all and keep her grades up. She had grown artistically talented over the years. Her art drawing for a school project was hung up in the school cafeteria for most of the school year. She was so excited when she was able to finally bring it home. She smiled from ear to ear, skipping up to the house. She couldn't wait to show it off.

Ashley grew up so fast. She was wise beyond her age and taller, too. By the time she was 13, she was 5 feet 10 inches. I can't remember ever sharing clothes with her. She never wore my sizes. She would always tease me as she towered above me about how short I was. She had her own style, always wearing jeans, usually with a t-shirt.

I remember you loved your Vans, special skater sneakers. You had them in purple and black. You'd beg all the time to wear your slippers, though they were your favorite choice. You'd usually wear long necklaces with charms dangling from them. You hated wearing a coat. You'd say it wasn't comfortable. You loved wearing your Oregon Ducks sweatshirt and flip-flops. You were very kick back and chill. Dresses and skirts were not your style. You loved flashy loud belts with lots of rhinestones. To be silly, you loved wearing thick black glasses without their lenses. They had a square shape too them. You loved to take pictures wearing them. They gave you lots of attitude and style, you'd say.

Like most teens Ashley had also acquired a liking for Monster Energy drinks and caramel blended coffee. I didn't care for her drinking either one.

Ashley was always a big help everywhere she went. It was her natural instinct to help out and play with her younger siblings and cousins. They all adored her and looked up to her. Ashley began helping me with my detail cleaning business when she was about 12. She was a hard little worker. She always learned quickly and was always willing to help. We were able to grow even closer with her working with me. She was my favorite helper. I hoped one day she would want to take over for me, but she always said, "I'm going to be a marine biologist when I grow up." She wanted to move to Hawaii where she could study oceanography. She had a big love for the ocean and dolphins.

Ashley loved playing games, whether it was wall ball and basketball outside, or cards and dice with me inside on a rainy day. She was very competitive but had good sportsmanship. She was also very silly. One day during the winter when it snowed, she made a mini snowman about a foot tall and decorated it. She surprised me by placing it in the freezer. I took a picture of it. I thought it was very sweet of her.

Sometimes, she wasn't funny. On the weekends she liked to sleep in just long enough for me to do the dishes. Then she would conveniently come out of her room. She thought she was so clever. I never really minded though. I liked keeping the house all in order for her and our family. Other than cleaning her bedroom, she rarely had to do any house chores. When things were tough at home and there wasn't much in the cabinets to eat or we were in need, she would never complain. She kept a positive attitude and kept her head up. She knew having an attitude about the situation we were in was not going to help. She never wanted to make us feel bad. She knew how hard we worked to provide for our family.

For fun, Ashley, Mariah and I used to love to eat out at China Hut. This was her favorite restaurant. She loved it. We loved walking the mall and window shopping. Deb and Aeropostale were her two favorite stores. We'd always watch the chick flick movies together. Rachel Mc Adams was her favorite actress. We loved her movies—they always made us cry. In the truck, we would crank up the stereo real loud. We loved listening to Jason Aldean and Luke Bryan. As a family, we always enjoyed going to Ashland. We would walk through Lithia Park and she would play on the playground with Mariah. She loved going to the chocolate store downtown in Ashland. We would all pick out a candy and window shop. At night when we lived in Grants Pass, we would go to the fairgrounds. We'd sneak in through the back where the fencing was broken. The horses were back there in the stalls, dozens of them. The girls loved walking around petting all of them. It was so peaceful and quiet at night.

Our biggest vacation as a family was when we went to visit Justin's grandma, Rainy, in Modesto, California. We were able go over to the Raging Waters water park in Sacramento. The kids had so much fun, we spent the whole day there. The rest of the time was spent visiting family and swimming in Grandma's pool.

We went on lots of other family trips. One of her favorite trips was when all the family went to the Whale's Head cabins at the beach in Brookings, Oregon. We spent three days up there and the kids all took over the hot tub and the T.V. They all remember that trip!

We spent many summers at my parents' place visiting. Ashley loved swimming in the creek with her younger cousin, Erin. Erin was just a year younger and they got along great. At night, we'd have bonfires and sometimes camp out. She was close with most of her cousins who lived around us. She was like a sister for some of her male cousins. During my last trimester, when I was pregnant with Ashley, her older cousin, Jeremiah, would sit on my lap and rub my belly. He would talk to Ashley and tell her he loved her. He couldn't wait for her to be born. From the first day he met her he always had a special bond with her. He was only a year old when she was born and he loved her already.

All the cousins confided their secrets to Ashley and trusted her. She was always fun and never controlling. She seemed to be the mediator amongst them. She always kept things under control when they'd get together. For years they were all able to visit on a weekly basis. We were always hanging out. Especially around the holidays, we made sure they were special each year for the kids. The family was always getting together for good times.

When we moved from Grants Pass back to be Medford area, Ashley was 10. This was Ashley's favorite place we lived in. It just happened to be on the street next to her favorite cousin, Nessie. Ashley and Nessie would always take their dogs on walks together around the neighborhood. Nessie's dog, Honey

Bear, was the daughter of Ashley's dog, Sadie. The four of them loved their walks together.

Around this time, Ashley started 6th grade at Scenic Middle. She quickly made friends in this school. It was easier there because lots of kids lived in our neighborhood. She would take Mariah down to the park with her dog Sadie all the time. Usually there would be kids from close by and she liked playing basketball and tetherball. Soon Ashley met a very good friend of hers and they began spending nights at each other's houses. They had goofy nicknames for each other. During one of their sleepovers, they took a basketball and passed it back and forth, each writing silly notes on it. They called each other "Cheese burger" and "Mc Nugget". Ashley started attending a church close by with her Aunt Bobbi and family. For the couple of years, we lived there she was able to attend most Sundays. It was very hard for her when we had to move again. She had met many friends there that she loved and adored. She begged us not to move out of her school district. Unfortunately, the house we found was out of the district. We chose this place because we had the opportunity to buy it. We were tired of having to move every few years and wanted something of our own.

We moved in October of 2010 out to Eagle Point. Ashley struggled her first year. We had to move in the middle of her school year. This puts all eyes on you when you are starting a new school in the middle of the year. She was so self-conscious, she started worrying about fitting in. The kids out here in our small town mostly grew up together and their groups were all formed. It took her awhile to find her right group, kids that she felt comfortable being herself with.

She met a friend and was soon being invited over after school and on weekends. Their family completely adored Ashley. They were also a goofy, fun, down-to-earth bunch. Eagle Point is small, so on Friday night kids in town liked to gather at Campus

Life. This was the community building in town specifically for teens. They have adult supervision there so we didn't have a problem with her going.

Ashley began making other friends and soon she was always asking to do something. She had a friend she began to grow very close to who lived down our street. They were always being crazy, having fun. They would push each other around in the shopping carts at Wal-Mart. Or dress up in ridiculous outfits and walk through town just to see people's reaction.

Ashley and Mariah loved walking with me. We liked to walk on the path leading around the golf course. At the beginning where we parked the car there was a bakery. We loved to get a doughnut before the walk. Across from the golf course were pastures. We loved to feed and pet the horses. We were always spending time together. Ashley was Mariah's best friend and my best friend. She was irreplaceable.

At the beginning of our 2nd summer living in Eagle Point, we were able to buy an above-ground swimming pool. It was dark outside before we got back home. Justin and Ashley and Mariah were so excited they stayed up till 1:00 am putting it together. They probably spent at least 5 hours working on it. Took all night to fill, but in the morning when they woke, it was ready. Ashley and Mariah spent the whole summer that year in that pool. We were surprised they didn't turn into fish. The pool definitely made a lot of good memories. That summer, T. J. got his driver's license, so for his 16th birthday we gave him the Mustang we'd been driving. Ashley thought it was so awesome being able to ride with him. She couldn't wait for them to be able to go hang out alone.

That year in November I signed a large contract detail cleaning 46 apartments. They took three months to complete. Ashley worked there with me the whole time. She would help on weekends and after school she loved earning money. When the project was complete she had earned enough to buy herself an Xbox360 Kinect with three games. She was so proud of herself we were proud of her too.

Ashley turned 14 years old that year, in 2012. She seemed to be going on 16 though, always trying to grow up so fast. We were always pulling back on the reins, slowing her down and telling her, that she could wear her make-up lightly but she wasn't allowed to date boys. Her time was spent with family and friends. She was always trying to tease and trick us all. She had one friend that spent the night with who she had believing Taylor Swift had signed her guitar. Of course Ashley had signed Taylor's signature herself. She was so amused with herself. She was always entertaining for her friends and family to be around.

I had been working a lot and we could afford to relax. I wanted to surprise Ashley and do something she always dreamed of. So I took Ashley by herself to the mall. I was able to spend a few hundred dollars on her for clothes and she was super-excited. She was able to go into any store she chose and shop. She bought half a dozen outfits that day. She was in Heaven; she couldn't quit thanking us. It felt good to be able to do that for her.

Ashley never bragged about what she got. She was always very humble. When the kids came back from Christmas break, Ashley told us that some kids didn't get anything. That year we had been able to spoil her rotten. She never bragged. She didn't want to make the kids feel bad. That was our Ashley, so sweet and humble. She was always thinking of others and their feelings.

There was a time when our mailboxes out front had fallen down. The wood was old and unstable. Our elderly neighbor was out front trying to lift the mailbox and fix it. He was struggling and there across the street were two middle-aged men capable of lending a hand. Neither even bothered to ask him if he needed help. Ashley was at home that day with Mariah and she watched this happen through the window. She knew he needed help so she and Mariah went out front to lend a hand. She was so sweet. When her great grandma passed a few years back she kept her nightgown folded in her dresser drawer.

Ashley was becoming a sweet and beautiful young lady, so intelligent and respectful, always concerned for others. She blossomed into a young woman right before our eyes. Her hair grew longer and she had such big beautiful brown eyes. Her hands were long and slender. She always had long nails—never had a problem growing them out. Her skin always looked tan. She had a natural glow to her. Her self-confidence was starting to show and we could tell she liked herself. She held her head high and proudly.

Things were going good. Ashley felt she was finally fitting in. We had no plans to move and she began to feel at home in Eagle Point. She spent time with friends and seemed socially content. She stopped asking to go back to her old school. We were happy for her and things seemed to be working out for her. So when she was invited to a slumber party for a friend's birthday we said "yes." We felt confident in our decision. She had spent nights before with this friend. The friend only lived five minutes away, and Ashley always checked in. Ashley never got into trouble. She was always a good kid, so we never worried too much. She made good decisions and knew right from wrong. She never got in trouble, not with us or her teachers, and never with the police. We were super proud of her.

The Day of the Slumber Party

O N THE DAY of the slumber party, Ashley woke up in the best mood. She was so excited to be able to go. That morning she spent extra time with her sister doing her hair for her. Justin, her stepfather and she spent time playing on the Xbox game system she had bought with her hard-earned money. She loved that game. She would have dance-off competitions with her sister and friends. That morning she weighed herself and realized she had lost 5 pounds. She had only had the game for a month or two. She saw that by dancing and having fun she was also exercising and trimming up. She had us take a picture of her. She wanted to keep track of her progress. In the picture, she is standing sideways and smiling ear-to-ear, with her stomach completely showing, and she never showed her stomach. She was so excited that she gave her dad Allen and the family in Washington a call. She told them how she had lost the weight. She told them she loved them. She added that she would see them soon as she hung up the phone.

Ashley's Grandma Debbie was planning to take her up there for a visit. It had been quite a while since her last visit. Around 2:00 that afternoon, she got her things and said goodbye to us, preparing to go visit her friend. She stood in our entryway in front of the door. We gave her a hug and said, "Love You." We told her to call around 6:00 pm that night to check in. She was headed down our street to meet up with another friend invited to slumber party and they were going to finish getting ready. When 6:00 pm came around, Ashley did call and check in. I asked her how things were. She said everything was fine; that they were having fun. I thought nothing was out of ordinary. I could hear the girls in the background. Everything seemed as planned.

The Call

I WOKE UP TO a phone call around 10:45 pm that night. There was an officer from the Medford PD on the other end. He told me paramedics were working on my daughter, that we needed to come straight to the hospital. They would meet us there.

I was paralyzed, stunned. I told him "no," that my daughter was here in Eagle Point at a teenage slumber party. He must be mistaken, but he was calling from Ashley's friend's phone. He then said again that he was with Medford police and asked whether Ashley Long was my daughter? I said "yes" and told Justin we had to go now. Something was wrong with Ashley and the police weren't giving more info. We live 15 minutes from Medford and that ride to the hospital felt like 2 hours.

When we arrived at the hospital, we were met by staff who directed us to a small counseling room. We were so confused. Why hadn't they taken us directly to see Ashley? Minutes went by and finally a doctor came in with staff. The words he said echoed through the room, "We have a very serious situation."

They then began to tell us that Ashley had suffered from asphyxiation. She had inhaled helium from a pressurized tank and collapsed. When the helium went into her lungs, it sent air bubbles through her veins and into her heart and brain, causing significant damage which resulted in her death. In that instant a part of me died. Our life was forever changed.

After hearing of our daughter's sudden death we were left in a state of utter confusion. How did our daughter get to Medford? Why? What had happened in Eagle Point to change where the kids were supposed to be? Who were they with? Why hadn't the mother called to tell us plans had changed? All our questions would soon be answered.

An officer soon met up with us at the hospital and explained what had happened that night. Apparently the mother of the home where the slumber party was to be held felt ill. Between her and the daughter, it's not clear who suggested a family member of theirs would be a better place to have the slumber party. The event was then changed and this decision was made sometime before Ashley and her best friend got picked up. When the birthday girl showed up to pick up the two girls that was when Ashley realized that the plans were changed. The girls didn't know this 28-year-old woman who was now hosting their event. She was the sister-in-law to the birthday girl. She lived in a nearby town and she had not met the girl's parents prior to that night. Kids being kids, they just wanted to hang out and have fun. They were swept right up and went along with this change.

It turned out that this woman had another plan for their evening. She purchased the alcohol in our home town of Eagle Point. After picking up our daughter Ashley and the other girls. So when they got back to her house, she then proceeded to mix drinks for the kids and offer them marijuana. When Ashley was offered marijuana she said "know." However, she did drink alcohol. As if that wasn't enough, she then invited three of her friends who were grown men back to her house where they all started hanging out and drinking with the under-aged kids.

At some point, one of the men saw a helium tank that the

woman had in her house for her own kids to play with. They used it for a remote control flying fish balloon. The man started inhaling helium from the tank, which made his voice sound funny. He then passed the tank around to each of her friends. One by one they inhaled helium, laughing and talking funny. When Ashley was approached to try it, her friends say she was hesitant, standoffish. Then the man told her that "it's ok, it won't hurt you and your friends all just did it!" So she gave in to the pressure . . . . The man turned the valve on the tank and held the mask up to Ashley, according to her friends.

As soon as Ashley inhaled the helium she got light-headed and dizzy. She tried to say something but collapsed. Initially, her friends all thought she was playing. But when they realized she was unconscious, the adults kept the kids from calling 9-1-1. The woman instantly panicked and insisted that all alcohol was cleaned up first. Ashley's best friend immediately started trying to give her CPR. She couldn't get Ashley to respond. She started panicking. It has been said that almost 20 minutes went by before one of the kids dialed 9-1-1 and tossed the phone to the woman in charge. The whole time my daughter was lying on the ground unconscious and not breathing. Before the police arrived the older men left and the kids were schooled on what happened and what to say. The woman looked out only for herself that night. Leaving all the kids hanging, she denied her involvement. She wouldn't say how they got to her house and refused to admit to buying them the alcohol.

We couldn't believe what we were hearing. It was like being in a fog and everything stops around you. The doctor told us they needed someone to identify Ashley. So my father, Sister Brandi and Justin went in to see her. They kissed her forehead and told her how much we all loved her. I couldn't do it. I froze. I didn't want to see my beautiful baby girl lying their lifeless. Calls were made to family, my parents first. I was completely falling apart and needed them now. They couldn't get there fast enough.

Trying to get hold of people was impossible in the middle of night. Aunt Bobbi and Michelle were reached first and they came up immediately. We didn't know how to break the news to her father, Allen, so Michelle made the call to him. He started driving down from Washington that night. Professionals can be so cold and they forget that this might be the first time families may be experiencing death. Our world had just been train-wrecked and yet they carry on as if they are used to it. Leaving the hospital without her was devastating. I had to leave her at same place where just 14 years before I gave birth to her. It is almost impossible for your brain to rationalize when you have been so traumatized. My body went into shock that night. I experienced uncontrollable vomiting, and instant depression. Our home was blanketed with a dark shadow. It became a lifeless box, where we were stuck, frozen in time. Losing Ashley felt like we lost the color in our lives, our happiness that was so strong in our family.

Telling Brother and Sister

The night of the accident Ashley's sister Mariah had spent the night with her cousin. We didn't know how we were going to be able to tell her. She was only nine and never experienced a loss. We know this news was going to devastate her and change things forever. So we waited till the following day to tell her. During this time our cousin Steve took Mariah and her cousin Selena to the movies and the parl. He tried to give her a fun filled day before she was told the devastating news about her sister. We had gathered the grandparents and they would be support for all of us. We planned on telling her at home after picking her up. On the ride home she must have asked where her sister was three times and we kept distracting her changing the subject. It was heartbreaking. Ashley was her favorite person in the world they did everything together. She looked up to her so much. Telling her was the hardest thing to do. You could see her whole world crashing we watcher her heart break. She had so many questions. We told her that her sister had an accident and was now up in heaven. We explained how her and her friends had inhaled helium to sound funny. We explained how the helium hurt her and that it was an accident. That Ashely didn't know what would happen and that it wasn't her fault. Having our parents their helped all we could do was hold her and cry.

That weekend T.J. had gone camping so he was unreachable

for a few days. We were worried that he would hear about Ashely from the news or Facebook first. We did now want that to happen so we kept calling his phone. We could tell when he was getting closer to town or in range. His cell phone went from sending you straight to voicemail to now a static ring. When Justin was finally able to reach T.J. he first asked if he could speak to his mother Tally. Justin told Tally what had happened to Ashley that weekend and asked her to please be there for T.J. because he could not at the moment. Then T.J. got back on the phone and Justin explained what had happened to him. T.J. knew we needed him here so he drove up from California to be here during everything we were going through.

The First School Day Following

THAT FIRST MONDAY following the accident, Justin and Mariah gathered strength together. Justin wanted to gather Ashley's belongings and bring them home. So that morning, they went down to Ashley's school. As they were walking into the school, Justin could see that a grief counseling area had been set up for kids in the Library if they needed to talk. Justin went inside the Library with Mariah. Lots of kids were gathered. Justin was able to take that moment to talk about what happened to Ashley and warn the teenagers about the dangers of inhaling helium. He talked about peer pressure and how it affects others.

Then the Principal and a Pastor from a local church took a moment and prayed with Justin and Mariah. They went and collected Ashley's belongings from her lockers. The teachers told Justin how much they enjoyed having Ashley in their classes. The kids at school all began wearing purple in honor of her and a club was formed called "The Ashley Hope Club." The club focused on peer pressure and helium danger awareness. The girls in the club spent time making donation containers and placing them around our local town. These were in hopes of raising money towards awareness about helium. We had sweatshirts and t-shirts made, along with bracelets. The shirts had Ashley's Hope Awareness in purple and white printed on them. The girls worked hard and were heartfelt in their mission. Always positive and full of ideas. We were proud of them and grateful.

Receiving Final Documents

W E RECEIVED HER death certificate the following week in the mail. Why it's a "certificate" I'll never understand. A certificate is usually an accomplishment, something positive. There is nothing positive about a death certificate. It's a piece of paper that came in the mail announcing the death of our daughter. I hated that piece of paper. I wanted so badly to rip it into a million pieces.

It took a couple of weeks for the autopsy results to come back. They showed .04% alcohol level and no marijuana in her system. That last morning with Ashley, we were in the kitchen at breakfast and the discussion about marijuana came up. She told us that she would never try it. She stayed true to those words. We are so proud of her for that. When her friends were all gathered around smoking, she chose not to. That being said, she did inhale the helium against her better judgment. Tragically this decision cost her her life. The adult in charge had given her and her friends alcohol, which impaired her judgment. Ashley wasn't looking to get high that night. She did want to laugh with her friends, however, and have fun, like a typical teenager. My daughter died laughing. This is devastating. As a parent, I close my eyes and I can still see Ashley laughing and smiling.

The Funeral

NO PARENT CAN ever be prepared for the emotions and trauma following a child's sudden death. One moment you're planning their future with them, asking what they plan to be. And the next you're planning their funeral. No one can prepare you for picking out your child's coffin or for picking out their last outfit. How do you choose where she will be placed in the earth when her family is all still living? There are no do-over's; these decisions are final. Everything feels like it's spinning out of your control.

The funeral arrangers are so corporate and everything has to be paid up-front financially. They walk you through the grounds like you're picking out your vacation site. It's devastating the whole time. I remember when we were making the arrangements, we sat at a table and when it came time to choose a coffin, they had a room divider directly behind us. I remember the loud sound the divider made when they pulled it open. My heart broke again. Instead of picking out a prom dress or our daughter's first car, we were faced with the nightmare of planning her funeral.

We held her funeral on Sunday February the 26th. There was a beautiful clear blue sky that day. It was very cold outside and the wind was blowing slightly. So many loved ones showed up to pay their respects and say goodbye that day. The whole day is partially a blur. I don't remember getting ready for the service. I can remember arriving to the funeral home and family and friends meeting us outside. When we went inside to attend the service, there was an ocean of people.

All of your family and friends were there, Ashley. Many of your teachers attended the funeral home. It was overflowing with loved ones. They were all there for you. I remember feeling weak and trembling as Justin and I walked together with Mariah and T.J.

We all walked towards Ashley, holding hands. She laid there so peaceful, like Snow White. We kissed her forehead and told her we loved her. It felt like a dream, like all she needed was a kiss to wake her. That didn't happen though. She wouldn't wake up. I remember how cold her body felt, and when I tried to hold her hand it was stiff. This was the only time I saw her in this condition, and it was heart-breaking.

I brought one of the tiny Eiffel towers I collected and wanted to place it with you. I remember I couldn't open your hand, so Justin tucked it inside your palm for me. Each of us wrote you a letter expressing how you changed our lives for the better. How much you meant to our family and how much we'd miss you. We placed them inside your casket next to you. Your Uncle Rob bought you a diamond necklace that we placed around your neck. Many of your cousins had special items that they also placed with you.

When the service began, we had chosen "If I Die Young" and "I Hope You Dance" to be played during the ceremony. Both of your dads had written something special they read out loud. They were so strong. I had so much to say, so much love to express, but I was too emotional and fatigued to speak. I couldn't believe where we were and what we were doing. My mind didn't want to accept it. It was all happening in front of me and yet it was like being trapped in a nightmare. I just wanted to wake up.

After the ceremony we held a wake at the Grange in Eagle Point which all our family and friends were invited to attend. When we arrived, the kids from school had giant poster boards all around the building. They had all signed and written things to you, Ashley. They wrote how much they loved and missed you. Some wrote how you inspired them. They described about their first time meeting you. Others wrote about a special memory they had with you. They all had something nice to say.

We stayed at the wake about two hours and came home again without you. That is very hard to accept. We go home now every night and you're not coming home. Now all we have are memories and a lock of your hair. Your headstone I designed myself, choosing a large butterfly with the words, *"The light of your life will forever live on in our hearts. You were a wonderful daughter and we will always love you."* There are two tiny butterflies on the left-hand side and on the right lower side is a picture of Ashley. The writing is all done in purple ink. At the time yours was the only headstone on the grounds with color. That's how we remember you, always standing out being the leader. You were the brightest one.

Her stepfather wrote her a poem, using our nickname for her, Ashers.

Justin's poem

Oh Ashers so beautiful so sweet
We all love you so much
We are not sure how it will be
Without you tomorrow,
Next, month or year
One thing I do know

There will be many tears
From all of our family
And all her peers
She touched all our hearts
That's why we are in tears.
Oh sweet Ashers
You were so funny and smart
Thank you for the memories
You've etched in our hearts
Your brother and sisters
Who love you so so much
Will remember you forever
And forever they'll love
Oh amazing Ashley
Oh what can we say?
Jesus is the only lucky one today
Oh sweet Jesus how lucky you are
To have our little angel
To do all your art.
I just want to tell you
How sweet she really is
In case you missed something
Up in heaven above
She helped little girls
who might not have been
Girls who were broken
Without any friends
Oh sweet Ashers you were the
Kindest and sweetest little soul
Not only that, but you were really cool
Oh our precious Ashers,
Someday we will see
You up in heaven

Where there you will be.
Oh Lord I have just one wish
Please hold our baby
And give her a kiss.

Your forever loving Step Father J Man

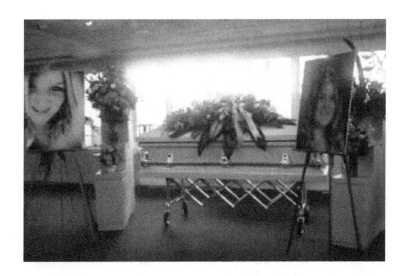

The Media

I
MMEDIATELY FOLLOWING ASHLEY'S death, the news channels all started calling. The next day she was in all the local papers and on all the news channels. The Associated Press came to our home for an interview. The media kept calling from all over. Ashley's story went national quickly. Losing your life to helium is rare and the public needed to know the dangers. Her story was soon on YouTube and all over the internet.

We were invited on the *Today Show* in New York after the funeral. They wanted to air our story. So, completely fatigued and heartbroken, we went to New York to attend the *Today Show*. We were determined to start spreading awareness about helium dangers. This was the hardest time my family had gone through and we were in no condition to travel but, for the chance to tell Ashley's story and prevent someone else from this tragic death, we had to go. Justin and I, my mother Connie, Mariah and T.J. all went. While we were in New York, we also went on The *Inside Edition* show. They had arranged for us to be able to tell Ashley's story and talk about helium. It was difficult having to tell the story so many times, but it is also very important we believe.

A week later we got calls inviting us to Washington, DC. There was a national inhalant prevention meeting scheduled. There were people from the press, and the entertainment industry and members of the White House staff that were attending. They asked us to be guest speakers, giving us a chance to tell people about the dangers of inhaling helium and our daughter's story. We attended that meeting as well, hoping to make a difference in Ashley's memory. Justin gave a-prepared speech he wrote during the conference. At the end of the meeting everyone approached us and thanked us for sharing. We believe that meeting was helpful in spreading awareness about helium. We are grateful for all the opportunities that we have been given to tell Ashley's story. Being able to spread awareness helps and gives our family something positive to focus on. This is a very tragic and devastating way to lose a loved one and it can be prevented by awareness.

Our Angles on Earth

DURING OUR FAMILY'S time of need, my mother was immediately there for us. She stayed with us for the first few months. She helped with everything from moral support to the daily household tasks. We were grateful to have her—she was our rock. There were many family members that were there for us. We never felt alone. They handled everything from setting up the different web sites to spreading awareness, to handling all of the media calls and questions they had. For several months, our house seemed chaotic. The phone was always ringing and appointments were being made left and right. Suddenly there were lawyers and legal matters to be dealt with. Family and friends were there through it all. We all wanted to do the best we could by Ashley.

In our community there have been a handful of families that have reached out, each helping in their own special ways. Many brought flowers and groceries and were full of condolences. Mariah's teacher came to the house after bringing her a giant monkey. Several families have invited us into their homes hoping to heal our hearts. We have shared our pain and they have listened, their hearts breaking for us. They all opened their doors and have a special place for Mariah in their families. We have been able to grow close with them during this difficult time. All of them have girls and this has given Mariah some new friends to spend time with. She felt alone without her sister and having friends helps her heal. Truly it has been a blessing, making it easier to stay in Eagle Point. These families hold a special place in our hearts. We will never forget their gratitude and kindness.

When the accident happened, the families of the kids involved moved out of our town, everyone except for us, making the town feel pretty lonely. After a tragedy like this, you feel like all eyes on you and your family. For months we had a hard time in public because of our story. The local news kept airing information about the case for the entire year until sentencing. People can be cruel and ignorant when uneducated. There were many people who argued about how Ashley died. They hadn't ever heard before that inhaling helium is deadly. It is rare but there are several cases on the internet. What kind of person argues with a parent on how their own child lost their life?

The Darkness Following

WHEN EVERYTHING HAD taken place and emotions sank in during the days that followed, our world became very dark. Your bodies shut down. You cannot physically work or function normally in your daily life. We were unable to work for months afterwards. Justin stayed home with me and never left my side. Things quickly fell behind. The bills soon started piling up. Justin and I have always been self-employed. We each have small businesses. With everything we were going through it was hard being social and finding new jobs.

The amount of anxiety that built up became unbearable. Your mind becomes your worst enemy, constantly trying to rationalize what it's been through. It was nearly impossible to get through each day. Minutes felt like hours; days felt like weeks. Everything I once found joy in was no longer there. Daily walks I once loved and window shopping. Taking a shower and getting dressed for the day became an overwhelming task. I just lay on the coach for months and cried every day. Tears would not stop flowing. They were uncontrollable. I felt numb to life. My world felt so empty. We felt like our family's happiness had been stolen.

I no longer even recognized myself without Ashley. I truly lost myself. I found myself constantly having to remind myself of my loved ones that were there and needed me. The pain just consumed me, and there were a few times when I didn't want to be alive. I didn't even want to think of spending the rest of my life without her. It hurt so badly she had been so healthy. There was nothing wrong with her. I had done nothing but plan for her future her entire life. Suddenly in an instant, it was over without a chance to say good bye. It wasn't fair. There are so many bad people in the world, and yet, the sweetest one gets taken.

I instantly hated my new home. I was full of regret for moving to this town. I kept going over and over in my head all of the what if's. I was so sorry we had moved there. If she hadn't had chance to meet this particular crowd, she'd still be here. Why did the next house we found have to be in Eagle Point? I had no desire to cook anymore. Cooking only reminded me that I needed enough for three instead of four now. Out of the four of us, Ashley was the one who ate like I do. Justin and Mariah don't like eating fruit and vegetables and Ashley and I love them. She also loved strawberry flavored things and cheesecake. Not Mariah and Justin—they love chocolate. I miss having someone in the house that shares my food likes. It can be a lonely feeling trying to make fruit and veggie dishes for just one. But then, everything seemed to hurt. I couldn't escape them.

There is a guilt that sinks in because you are still here and your child is gone. I couldn't physically eat. My body wouldn't allow me too. I had a hard time controlling my stomach. The only thing I was able to keep down the first month was Ensure. I hated being awake; it was unbearable. The pain I experienced from losing Ashley was excruciating. I felt as if a knife had gone straight through my heart and was still there. The one thing I needed to make it all go away was Ashley and she was forever gone.

So I slept for weeks and weeks. I prayed that I'd dream about

Ashley. I wanted so badly to be able to see her again, and hear her voice. It never happened. Night after night for some reason I couldn't remember dreaming anything. The moment I'd wake up before my head lifted from my pillow, my tears would be flowing like a faucet I couldn't turn them off. I never knew we could make so many tears. Everything and every place reminded us of her. Places we ate or shopped, they all felt empty. All the spots we went to as a family—they were everywhere around us. For the longest time, we didn't go anywhere. It was too painful.

Fortunately, Mariah found comfort instantly in drawing pictures and writing. She had a special table set up which she filled with things about Ashley. There were new gifts brought from friends and family along with Ashley's personal things from her bedroom. Mariah just wanted it close to her and all together. She would spend time looking at everything and putting all of Ashley's jewelry on. She slept with a picture of Ashley in an 8x10 frame for a few years. Since the accident, she was scared to be alone at night. She slept in our room on the ground floor every night for years. Each night before she falls asleep she always says, "Good night, Sissy," and, "I love you."

When your story becomes so public it makes you extremely self-conscious. We always felt like we were being watched or whispered about. It's another form of anxiety that builds up, controlling you. Your bus stop is a block from our home. Every morning I watch that bus drive by, wishing you were on it. When I see the kids walking home, I can still picture you holding your binder, smiling, walking in front of our house. I could always tell what kind of day you had before you even came through the door.

After you passed, we found things you had made. There was a disc in your computer you were working on right before the accident. It was for your dad and family in Washington. We were so surprised to find it. No one had seen it before. It felt like a gift left behind from you. The video was all about you and your favorite things, pictures of friends. You had pictures of family and all your pets included. It was so beautiful. We all gathered at the computer, watching and crying. Suddenly in the middle of the video you make us all laugh. You have a picture of you with two bobby pins in your mouth, making a silly face. It's my favorite one and this makes us all smile and laugh. It was perfect—just like you—always knowing how to cheer everyone up. We have found other surprises too. There was a Christmas note Ashley had made for me full of all the colors. I'd never seen it before. She wrote:

<blockquote align="center">
Mother Earp! Mother Earp! ☺
Merry Christmas I Love You!
You are amazingly awesome!
The best mom in the . . . world!!! ☺
Hope you have the best Christmas ever and
don't forget to get me something I'll love! ☺ ha ha
You are the best boss anyone could ever ask for!! Ha.
Someday I'm going to be the boss!! (:
And I love you!
—Ashley ☺ 2011
</blockquote>

The First Year
Without Ashley

W E HAVE CRIED now every day since you've been gone. There are reminders of you everywhere in our home. All the art you made in school and the Paris drawings you created. We have everything. We keep them safe and hold them close. The sticky notes you posted—you wrote, "*I heart mom*," still hang on the fridge. Learning to go on without you has been hardest thing we've ever done. Nothing is the same anymore and we are learning a new normal for our family.

It is now normal and part of life to visit Ashley at the cemetery. A place before we never had reason to be. Holidays are bittersweet without you and hurt in ways I can't describe. Every year for Easter, our family has a huge picnic and Easter egg hunt. There is a giant rock that all the kids gather around and we take a picture. You have always been there, but not this year nor any of the ones to follow.

This year my mother brought lots flat rocks and paint. All the kids and some adults painted a rock especially for Ashley. We placed them at the rock where we gather for the picture. This was our family's way of including her that day.

On Mother's Day, Justin surprised me with a drawing you had made but you never gave it to me. It was very special. I told him the day was really going to hurt because every year Ashley had made something special for me, usually in school. So it was so special to receive something from her even though she was gone.

When Christmas came around, the joy and happiness that always follows wasn't there. This was your favorite holiday. I couldn't decorate. So for Mariah, we got her a table-top Christmas tree and she decorated it. This way we were still celebrating the holiday. We didn't want to wake up Christmas morning without you, so as a gift, some friends of ours gave us a motel room in the next small town over. T.J. came up, which was super important. We didn't want Mariah to be the only one Christmas morning opening her presents. We brought the mini tree and the presents and spent the night at the motel.

When we arrived there was a German shepherd stray running around outside the motel. This caught our attention because that was Ashley's favorite type of dog. We began to unpack the truck and suddenly the dog ran into our motel room. It went and sat on the couch and just lay there. We didn't have the heart to kick it out. That dog stayed the whole night on the couch and in the morning, it went on its way. It was the strangest thing.

Your birthday came around in January. We had planned a memorial celebration at the cemetery for you. I ordered 70 purple sky lanterns that we released into the sky after singing "happy birthday" to you. All your friends and family were there. It was really beautiful, something I will always remember. At the end of the school year, your classmates all gathered in front of your school and planted a purple Rhododendron plant in your memory. In the yearbook, they had dedicated a page to you with your picture and the poem you wrote. Your friends and classmates all signed your book. The principal gave it to us at the tree planting.

It was hard knowing your classmates were moving on without

you. They would all be attending high school the following year. You had been anticipating high school your whole last year. You had so many questions. That first summer without you, to get through, we worked on our bare front yard. Everything we planted had you in mind. Every hole that was dug was for you. That summer we planted at least 50 plants and trees. Mariah and I found this to be very therapeutic. Turns out Mariah has a green thumb. Our yard looks beautiful.

Having to watch the kids on the bus start high school without Ashley stung my heart. She was robbed of so many precious moments, all her high school memories. The dances and going to all the football games with her friends.

You missed your first date with the boy you liked. Learning to drive and getting your first car. Graduating with all your friends. You would have been at the top of your class. They were all so excited to be starting this new chapter in their lives. Ashley should have been there. She deserved to be there. She had the biggest love for life and for everyone in hers.

Every morning I go into your room first thing and open your curtains. I want the light to shine through. I don't want your room feeling dark, ever.

Ashley's room is still full of everything she made and all her things. The jewelry she loved and wore remains in her jewelry box. Her school binder is still the way she left it on her last day of school. I kept her favorite clothes and tucked them away. The wall where she pinned all of her friends' notes and pictures are still there. When we turn off the light in her room, all you see is the glow in the dark doodles she made. They spell out thing like *sunshine* and *paradise*. There are smiley faces and *I Love You*. They seem to describe your personality. It's devastating to pass by your room every day and know you're not there. We miss the music we'd hear coming from your room and hearing you talking on the phone with your friends. We miss how warm and alive you made our home feel. Your laugh was something we heard almost every day of your life. We saw your beautiful smile every day. The longing urge I have to hug you never goes away. It grows larger with each day you are gone. I live with an ache inside me now and a world of regret.

Not long after she passed, we dug through some papers and found a note she had written. She was talking about how excited she was to be invited and going to the slumber party. She went on and on about how cool it was going to be. That it was her friend's birthday and she couldn't wait for that Saturday. She acted as if this was the event of a lifetime. This girl where the slumber party was supposed to be lived close to the golf course. Her house was fairly large and she had a hot tub. It was going to be so much fun and she was making friends, she thought. She never even saw it coming. Within a few hours her night had completely changed in direction. She went along with everyone and we had no knowledge of this taking place until after she has passed. We are left with a completely helpless feeling. Our daughter died amongst strangers.

I should have been there in her biggest time of need. I wasn't there that night and that haunts me still. Knowing that when she collapsed, I had no idea. I was at home in bed. It is so important to teach your children to always let you know where they are going and when plans change. That night I went to bed with no worries because I thought I knew where she was and what Ashley was doing. We were completely blindsided. Her night had spiraled so quickly out of control. She was just beginning to socialize in groups. I didn't realize alcohol was being introduced to some of her friends.

Kids these days experience life much earlier than we did due to the internet, I believe. It's so important to keep the communication and trust open between your children. When Ashley arrived that night at a place unfamiliar to her, I'm sure she was afraid to call home. She would have been scared because she wasn't supposed to be there. She wouldn't have wanted to let us down. So she went along with the night to fit in with all her friends. These are regrets I will live with for the rest of my life. I wish I had talked to her prior to that night and told her that no matter what situation she got into, she could always call home. That she didn't have to worry about getting into trouble—her being safe was the number one priority. I never got that chance.

There are haunting new dates throughout the year that we dread. January and February are our worst months. They hold Ashley's birthday and death anniversary. Anniversaries have always been a joyous occasion, something to look forward to. These are definitely not dates our family looks forward to. Her birthday breaks your heart more with each passing year. It is a reminder of what she lost and how much was taken.

When you love someone and take care of them for 14 years, it's almost impossible to wrap your mind around the reality that they are gone. They have no more laundry to wash or toiletries needed to be bought for them. When you cook for your family now, you need less. Shopping is disturbing. You can't help but see things all around that remind you of her. You hurt for everything she will miss out on. High school was something she was looking forward to—now she will never graduate. There will be no new pictures with her. She will never learn to drive and get her license. Never fall in love and get married. We will never know her as a mother or grandmother. She will stay forever young in our hearts and our pictures.

When we lost Ashley, we also lost a part of Mariah. Before her death, Mariah was the happiest little girl in the world. Nothing could break her spirit. She was full of life and love. Her heart had never seen pain. That all changed the instant we had to tell her about Ashley. It was devastating. Her world was upended forever in that moment. My heart hurt so badly for her. Ashley was her everything. We couldn't imagine her without Ashley by her side. Mariah has struggled in many ways over the past year to move on. It's been very hard for her to focus in school. Her mind is filled with so much that has happened at home. Justin and I have held Mariah close through this and together we make it through each day.

Each day we wake up with Ashley in our hearts and always on our mind. We share fond memories we had and always keep her pictures close. We have learned many lessons and never take life for granted anymore. We think carefully before letting Mariah spend time with others. I want to be sure that the adults in charge will treat her as they would their own, especially during an emergency.

We are so grateful for the times we live in. The technology has allowed for us to record so many precious memories. They each are like journals we have, holding Ashley's memories of her favorite things. Prior to Ashley's accident we had no interest in Facebook. I had never even seen it before this happened. I'm so glad we took the time to look into it. It has opened up a new way of communicating and sharing with family and friends. On Facebook we have been able to share and post with Ashley's friends since the accident. So many friends have posted very personal things on Ashley's page. From poems to stories of memories they have.

Your cousin Nessie posted on YouTube a video of her singing to you the song by Carrie Underwood, "*I will see you again.*" It should have been your 16th birthday and she dedicated the song to you. It has been very comforting and therapeutic for our family. Our family members created the Ashley Hope page and prior to the accident Ashley had a Facebook page. We are able to see our daughter through her friend's eyes and share pictures. I love when they post their stories and memories with Ashley. Many post how their feeling and we have been able to share with them. I can see that it makes a difference in their day. I know reading what friends have shared makes a difference in ours. It reminds us that she will never be forgotten and how much she was loved.

When summer ended and fall began, it was time for the school year to start. This was a difficult time for our family. Our lives needed to have some kind of normalcy and structure again. Our family became very sheltered and withdrawn from public places when the accident happened. It seemed everyone in our small town knew our story and who we were. Large crowds created a lot of anxiety for us. It didn't matter if they were groups of kids or adults. They all had either known Ashley or had heard about her story. So to avoid the crowds of people, Justin took Mariah to school and picked her up.

It was the second day of school and Justin was there picking Mariah up. The final bell letting the kids out of school had not rung yet. He was a few minutes early and all the parents were there waiting as well. He waited by the truck in the parking lot when another truck pulled in directly next to ours. A woman got out on the passenger side and Justin was sure he recognized her. He thought she was the person who had served alcohol to the kids at the party where Ashley died. He turned to the young man driving the truck she got out of and asked, "is that what's her name?" The young man didn't respond, so Justin walked on up to the school. He was sure it was her. You can't forget the face of the person who has changed your lives forever.

He could tell that the young man was immediately calling someone. The woman was now in front of the school standing alongside the other parents. All of a sudden, she walked directly towards Justin and asked him, "Are you looking for me?" The young man must have called her and given her a head's up that someone was looking for her. Justin was shocked that this woman didn't even recognize him. So he tells her, "You should know me, you killed our daughter." She immediately steps back and is completely uncomfortable. There are a lot of parents waiting out front and now all eyes are on them.

The woman begins saying she is so sorry about Ashley, how she never meant for anything to happen. Justin then explains to her in loud voice that our family had never seen any form of apology. Months had gone by and there had been nothing from the woman directly responsible for Ashley's death. He told her how broken we were and that I was at home devastated. He also told her he couldn't believe the nerve she had to enroll her kids in the same school as our younger daughter. Her kids didn't attend that school prior to the accident—they didn't even live in our town. They lived twenty minutes away, and yet she had enrolled her kids in our direct school district.

Justin told her that if that was the case and if she were truly remorseful then she shouldn't have chosen to put her kids in the same school as ours. She should have stayed as far away from us as she could out of respect. Our family had been through enough, and having to see and worry about running into her was too much. We lost our daughter because of her. We didn't want to be put through having to watch her drop off and pick up her kids on a daily basis. What was she thinking?

Our stories were still headline news on our local news channels and in all the newspapers. We were still waiting for her to be charged and sentenced. Our kids on either side didn't deserve to be put through that—they were innocent. The bell rang and the kids soon piled out. Justin didn't want Mariah to notice her so he quickly told her she disgusted him and walked away towards Mariah.

The woman kept her kids enrolled that whole year, making it impossible not to think about her. It was torture. Our town is so small that from the highway leading straight through it, there are only three roads she could choose to drive down when she drops her kids off at school. We live directly on the route she happened to take every day. She seemed to be like a magnet with us. If I were in her shoes I would have moved as far away as possible. That was how she acted during the whole 13 months that the courts took before they were charged. She kept being seen by our family and friends shopping at the mall or attending her kid's football games. We saw her a couple times in our local Wall-mart, and it was very hard having to be strong and walk away. We had to be patient and have faith that our justice system would take care of them. A system that time and time again we felt had let our family down. There was so much anger and anxiety that built up over that year. We lost our daughter directly because of her actions and yet she hadn't even spent one night in jail yet. The day Ashley died, I felt sentenced to my own prison. I was trapped in a nightmare that I could never escape.

Months went by and we suddenly got a call from the DA. It turns out that the woman had been arrested again for tampering with a witness in our case. She had been caught trying to coerce one of the kids involved. She was still causing damage. We needed the truth to come out and she was trying to conceal information. She was still looking out only for herself. We realized there was no way she was truly remorseful.

There were many questions we still had that were never answered. Did that woman plan on seriously dropping our kids off with hangovers the next day? Since she was a parent also, how could she think that was ok? They knew the moment they gave the girls alcohol they were wrong. That night Ashley's iPod was broken. We wonder how? This was her favorite thing and she was always careful. We wonder if there were pictures taken that night. So many teens and they all had cell phones with cameras. Ashley was always taking pictures—why not on that night? I'd like to be able to thank the child who finally gathered the courage to call 9-1-1. We don't know who made the call though.

I wonder what my daughter's last words and thoughts were. Was she in pain? Did she realize what had happened? These answers won't change anything—what's done is done. They would, however, bring some form of comfort just knowing what happened. I had hoped and prayed that the answers would all be told in court. That never happened though. Our case never went to trial. We never were able to hear the truth from the children themselves. It's cheaper for the county if they can offer plea bargains. They don't have to pay for drawn out trials.

The Sentencing

OVER A YEAR went by and the adults involved with her death finally were being charged. The 33-year-old man who brought the tank out was sentenced to 90 days in jail and a $10,000 restitution fine. He pleaded no contest to negligent criminal manslaughter. The woman was charged with providing alcohol and marijuana to minors. She was charged with criminal mistreatment in the first degree, meaning she kept Ashley from receiving medical attention when she collapsed. The woman was sentenced to prison for 28 months but was eligible for their programs allowing early release for good behavior.

That day was one of the hardest days of my life. I had to wait for over a year before they were sentenced and the anxiety that built up was overwhelming. I had so much I wanted to say to these complete strangers who were responsible for changing our lives. Neither one of them even bothered to try and apologize after a whole year. The courtroom was packed with our family and friends who filled the rows of seats. The local news channels and newspapers were standing along the wall. The DA and all the lawyers were up front, sitting at long tables. Justin and I sat in the first row directly behind the DA and all of Ashley's direct family sat behind us.

When the two people being sentenced walked in, they were

positioned next to the DA. So they were directly in front of us. My heart was pounding and I felt that fog come over me, like being trapped in a nightmare and you can't scream. I felt numb and weak, but I also knew this was our only day in court and I needed to be strong. The judge allowed us to speak, but we had to address him. Meaning we couldn't speak directly to them. They were who we were angry at, and I wanted them to have to face all of Ashley's family. I was able to hold up Ashley's lock of hair to show them. "This is all I have left," I told them crying hysterically.

The judge read them their sentences and we watched as they were handcuffed and taken into custody. Their time started immediately. It was a relief and a humbling feeling that we had waited so long for. We are angry about the outcome of our case though. We feel there should be harsher punishment for adults who party with minors. My daughter was a child. The woman had no right to treat her as an adult. There are reasons for age limits on alcohol. Both of the adults involved have young children of their own at home. I can't believe another parent would conduct themselves in this way. I will never know if they truly are sorry or realize the extent of what they have done. Our family will never be the same. This has affected us for rest of our lives.

We feel the justice system has let us down. We also feel the Helium Company should be held responsible for their product by warning people of potential dangers. I guess public safety is not one of their priorities—they are more concerned with making money. These charges did not feel like justice to our family. Ashley lost the rest of her life due to their irresponsible actions. She was only 14. Her whole life was still ahead of her. The other children involved will live with nightmare the rest of their lives. They had to watch their friend collapse and were stopped from calling 9-1-1. These images are forever etched in their minds. They can't change anything or run from the past. Just like our family, they have to learn to live with this and go on with their lives. That is exactly what Ashley would want. She would want the best for everyone. She would want you to live your life to the fullest. For you to be the best person you could be. She would not want the fact that she lost her life to destroy others.

Spreading Awareness on Helium

HELIUM BALLOONS ARE all around us every day. We buy them for our loved ones on every occasion. They are in stores hanging by strings within the reach of children. They are at the party you or a loved one is attending. People love to decorate using them. They are bright and colorful, inexpensive and look so inviting. Weddings, birthdays, baby showers, Prom—there are many reasons to celebrate. Balloons seem to be the number one choice for decorating. These balloons are usually filled with helium. There are many children's toys requiring helium—for instance the Air Swimmers flying balloon fish and sharks. There are helium filled bouncy balls called The Sky Ball. Or the helium-filled remote control saucer toy.

To fill these up, a pressurized tank is needed. These tanks are dangerous and should be kept away from children. People don't realize that when you inhale helium, you risk losing your life. Whether inhaling from a balloon or from the tank itself, this gas is deadly. There are several cases on the internet involving both types of death. It doesn't matter how many times you have tried it. You have no warning signs when helium expands inside you and pushes your oxygen out of lungs, filling them with helium. You can't survive only on helium. Your body requires oxygen or you will collapse.

Since our daughter's death, we have researched the internet and found several cases of people dying, not only from the use of a helium tank but also from helium balloons. When you inhale all the helium quickly out of a balloon, it has the same effect as the tank. The helium expands inside your lungs, pushing all the oxygen out, filling lungs with helium. Our lungs can't breathe with helium. We require oxygen. This causes asphyxiation to set in, resulting in death. People need to be aware that the gas inside is lethal and can hurt you. There is actually a restaurant that has helium on their menu. When ordered, you are brought a helium-filled balloon on a platter! Are they serious? They have no idea how dangerous this is. Next time you are in a situation where someone is attempting to inhale helium to make their voice change, please stop them. Let them know the dangers that are hidden. Give them the chance our Ashley never had.

I wish we had known sooner about helium. If I'd seen something on the dangers ahead of time, maybe I could have saved her. I would have passed my knowledge on to her. I would give anything to have that chance to warn my daughter. My wish now is that one day the helium companies will be forced to warn the public of the dangers with their product. It seems though that helium is still being taken lightly and used for advertising and in many movies for entertainment. If you go on the internet, dozens of videos come up teaching how to inhale and showing people doing it. All the people are laughing and seem to be having time of their life. What you rarely see are the stories and pictures of the people who died this way.

The Poison Control Center is not required to report deaths due to helium. This is misleading to the public and I feel this needs to be changed. New laws need to be passed changing the rules and regulations concerning the helium companies. They need to be required to publicly make people aware of the dangers of inhaling helium. They need to start teaching people not to inhale their product. They would still profit because people love balloons. But by being safe about their product and educating people, companies would be assets in the awareness, thereby saving lives. There are helium suicide kits you can buy online. They come in the mail. These kits are extremely accessible. Anyone can purchase them and they come complete with instructions.

Why aren't the helium companies being held more accountable? Their product sits on the bottom shelf in stores and these tanks have no child safety locks on the nozzles. The box should look like it contains poison with extra-large warnings. They are labeled, "keep out of reach of children," and yet a child can purchase these tanks with no questions asked. A baby can crawl up to one sitting on the floor for a party and within a couple of seconds put their mouth on the nozzle. This instantly releases the helium gas when the slightest amount of pressure is applied. We need to educate our loved ones and teach kids that helium is deadly. People can still decorate and enjoy balloons. We just need to stop chasing the silly voice that sounds so funny. There is nothing funny when you lose a loved one over laughter.

Since our daughter's passing I have created a Helium Awareness page on Facebook. On Pinterest there are Helium awareness pins I've made. Ashley's Grandma Valerie has spread awareness through Geocaching. This is a scavenger-type game that you do online and then physically find things hidden. She hid a few of the pins inside with the item and Ashley's story. Some of her Geos have made it across the country with people traveling.

I have found that in our family's efforts to spread awareness we have difficulties finding information about this subject. There just isn't much out there to educate the public about the dangers of inhaling helium. There don't seem to be any books on helium awareness. When you search YouTube or Google on the internet plenty of people all ages inhaling helium show up. Inhaling helium is like a game of Russian roulette. No one knows which one is their last breath when inhaling the gas. A butterfly is how her family imagines Ashley, now so beautiful and free. Purple represents the color her friends think of because she loved to wear purple Vans. They showed her stand-out bright personality. Ashley died in February and purple is the color for that month. It is for these reasons that I chose a purple butterfly to represent Helium Awareness.

Getting used to the media and being in the public eye was something our family had to learn about quickly. We were soon on T.V. and doing interviews following Ashley's death. In our hopes of spreading awareness, we have had to share Ashley's story time and time again. In the beginning, I struggled with this. I couldn't get through the whole story without breaking down and losing it. Justin was very helpful and almost always on cue, he knew when to step in and finish for me. Each time we told Ashley's story, we got stronger and felt more empowered. We could tell we were making a difference. Ashley was making a difference. It brings a humble feeling to our family knowing Ashley could be saving lives. Out of our family's tragedy something positive could come. We had a chance to take Ashley's story and turn it around to help others. We could prevent another family from going through this. We want Ashley to always be remembered, never forgotten. I hope one day that Helium will be on the list of dangers that our schools teach kids about. I hope the helium and balloon companies create public awareness commercials warning about inhaling dangers.

Our family continues to warn people every chance we get. When we are out in public and see someone with a tank or bundle of balloons, we try and use the opportunity to warn them about the hidden danger. When we come across a new story or new information, we share it with others. You can accomplish great things just by word of mouth. We can make a difference and we will. Ashley's story is just one of dozens that involve accidental deaths from helium. If you search the internet you will find many others. Whether accidental or by suicide, they all resulted in death. Unfortunately, this gas is costing lives and awareness is important.

Pictures in our efforts to raise awareness on helium dangers

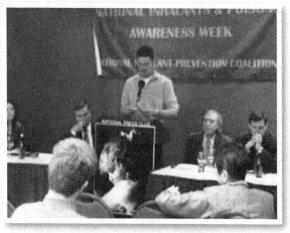

Justin Earp in Washington D.C. at the National Inhalant
Poison Prevention Coalition Week for 2012.

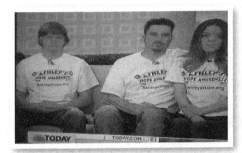

The Earp Family on The Today Show in
New York raising awareness.

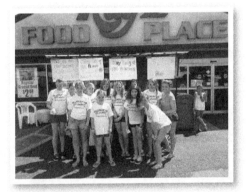

Ashley's Hope Club.

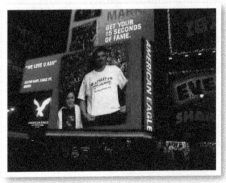

Justin and Mariah in Times Square, New York

Ashley's Grandma Valerie found another way to help raise awareness about helium dangers. She started Geocaching, which is a scavenger hunt game on the internet where you find Travel Bugs. You replace what you found with something similar for next person to find. She included Ashley's story about helium with her Travel Bugs. Currently there are six Travel Bugs with Ashley's story traveling around the world.

They were hidden and started from Medford, Or.

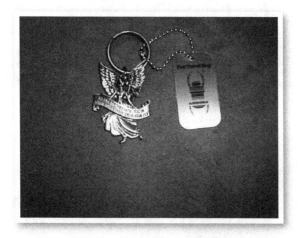

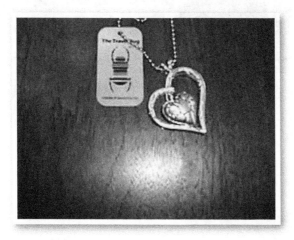

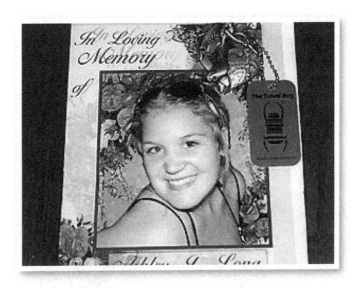

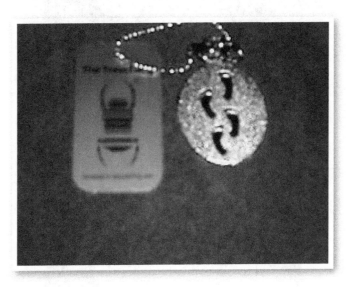

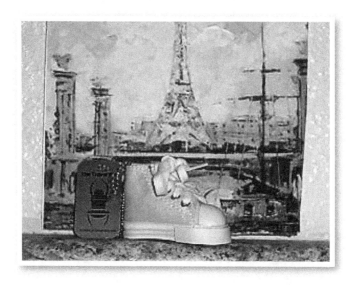

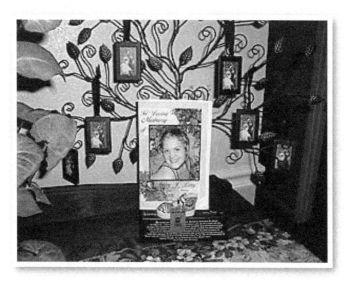

Alternatives to
Using Helium

THERE ARE MANY ways you can decorate using balloons without using helium. For instance, they make balloon sticks, allowing you to make balloon bouquets. These sticks also allow your balloon to stand up. You can hang them upside down with strings from the ceiling and in doorways. This makes a cool party effect. You can also make a homemade mixture of vinegar and baking soda inside a plastic water bottle. Then place the balloon over the mouth hole of the bottle and the balloon will fill up. This mixture creates a natural gas allowing balloons to float. Instead of a helium balloon, you can use different types of sky lanterns.

In writing this book I hope to educate people on the dangers of inhaling Helium. Ashley wasn't trying to get high with her friends. She just wanted to make her voice sound funny. No one should lose their life trying to laugh. Please help me spread awareness about Helium

This book is dedicated to the Memory of Ashley Jean Long
My loving daughter, our sweet angel in Heaven

Ashley's favorite things

#21 & #5 Purple VANS Color BLUE Peace tea Xbox I pod milk duds Peanut M&M's Oregon Ducks Zebra print Hawaii Dolphins The Ocean Chevy's 5 chewing gum Spaghetti Twilight Justin Bieber Transformer movies peace signs ☺ Hot Tamales All Music Camping Christmas watermelon Peanut Butter Hersey's Wall Ball Fashion Sponge Bob Butterflies Cheetos Slippers Whopper malt balls Mint chocolate chip ice cream Scary movies Hibiscus flowers Family Her pets swimming photography Her Friends Horses

MOST IMPORTANTLY SHE LOVED LAUGHING!!!

In Ashley's own words

When you think of me I'm sure these qualities
pop into your head.
Confidence, Strong, Positive, Believer, Faithfull, Artistic,

When I set a goal I reach that goal. I like completing my work on time so there's no worries. When it comes to a bad situation I don't give up I work it out never let myself down. Help others when needed and let them know when they did a good job. Drawing and listening to music are my two favorite things to do. I put my heart into my drawings. I like listening to country music because it reminds me of my life.

I am the one who ...

I am the one who loves to listen to all types of music . . . .

I am the one who enjoys spending time with my amazing friends . . .

I am the one who loves to watch funny movies . . .

I am the one who enjoys every minute of my life I can . . .

I am the one who loves making other people laugh and smile . . .

I am the one who loves playing sports . . .

Ashley's fun facts about herself

I AM CREATIVE, ARTISTIC, and outgoing, that's me! I always try my best to make people proud. I never give up no matter the situation. "Never say Never," that's what I live up to. This keeps me going and can lead to amazing things in your life that you can accomplish. I would love to be a photographer for a famous magazine. I love taking pictures and see things differently than people.

Family Letters to Ashley

A Letter to my Daughter

Dear Ashers,

I want to thank you for being so wonderful. You made it so easy to be proud of you. It broke my heart losing you and I'll never be the same. I feel truly blessed to have you as part of my life. You made all the colors brighter and the sun shine warmer. You brightened all our days with your smile so sweet. I will cherish all my memories and all that you made. I wish I could have taught you more and shown you the world. You taught me to love unconditionally. To also look out for and help one another. You taught me to stay true to my word and always be myself. You made my life so meaningful. Thank you for choosing me to be your mother. So glad you were in my life. You deserved to be treated like a princess and I will forever miss you. I know one day I'll see you again there you will be amongst the angels above.

I Love and miss you every day always & forever,

Your, Momma ☺

A Letter to my Sister

If you were here today I know what we'd be doing. You would be braiding my hair or we would be drawing. I miss swimming at the lake and playing wall ball with you. You'd be playing hide and seek with me and T.J. in the dark trying to scare me. I miss hanging out with you and your friends. Listening to music and playing the Xbox with you was so much fun. I loved playing dress up and taking pictures with you. I wish I could hug you and hear your voice again. When I call your name I wish you would come.

You were the best sissy ever I miss you!

Love, your sister Mariah

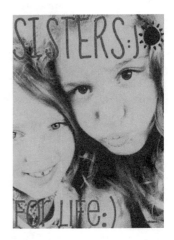

To all Ashley's family and friends with love

This book is a gift for all of Ashley's family and friends. In reading this I hope you share her story with future generations to come. I hope you always remember and never forget how she lived and how she died. Please be safe with helium.

R.I.P. Ashley Jean Long

Born Jan, 9th 1998 Died Feb, 18th 2012

Our sweet angel dancing in heaven ☺

Letter's from friends with love

A Letter from Cheyenne

I remember my dear friend from first and second grade. She had a contagious smile, glittering eyes and a shining smile. ☺ She always made me laugh. She had such a bright personality. I remember playing wall ball on the playground a lot with her. She broke her arm in first grade. I remember signing it. She'd let us punch her cast as hard as we could. Not realizing it hurt us more than her she was so funny. There will forever be a place in my heart that holds a bit of ash (:

Your loving friend,

Cheyenne

Right Beside Me

February 18, 2012.
She got her wings and her halo,
She's flying young wild and free;
Up there in heaven,
Shes still right beside me.

The helium was supposed to be a game.
Now you're set in the ground with a stone and your name,
With dates chiseled in,
Bringing me back again.

Being with you isn't the same.
Sitting 6ft below and I have so much to say.
I hope you hear these words today.
Why are you so far away?
How did God know you were the one to take?
I'm still waiting for him to admit, he made a mistake.

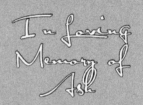

I'm Loving
Memory of
Ash

It took me a year to visit you,
I couldn't wrap my head around it.
I still can't believe you're not here,
Going on three years.
Through all these tears I wish you were still here.

All I know is;
I gotta pick myself up,
Catch my tears,
I'm being strong,
'Cause I know with every step I take,
Wild and free.
You're right beside me.

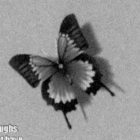

I'll remember your name,
The memories as they come,
Your story – a million to one.
Ashley's Hope, that's what we say
And it spreads awareness day by day.

Through the memories the tears the visits and the laughs,
Through the years that are to come and the years that have
passed.
You're young wild and free,
Right beside me.   —C. Lopez 2014

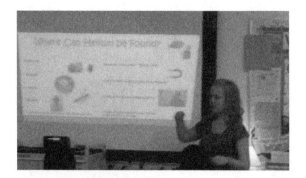

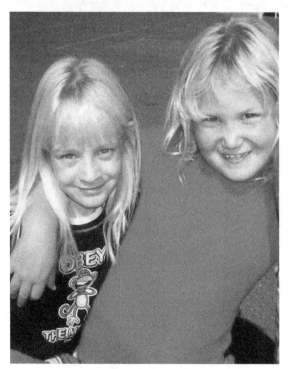

Cheyenne (left), Ashley (right).

A Letter from Taylor

The last time I saw you we were hanging out. You asked me to sing "pray" by Justin Bieber. We both started laughing. It was a moment I'll never forget.

Love, Taylor

A letter from Emily

Ashley was my most favorite person ☺. She was my Mc Nugget and I was her Cheeseburger. One time at her house we were eating Doritos and I started choking. She didn't believe me at first and started laughing. She soon figured it out and from then on was my superhero.

Love your "cheeseburger",

Emily

A letter from Alexis

I 'll always remember 5th grade. We jammed together listening to the song *Miss Independent* real loud. It was so amazing looking back on it.

<3 I miss her much love <3

Alexis

Pictures and Memories of Ashley's life

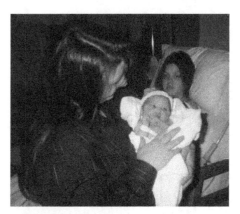
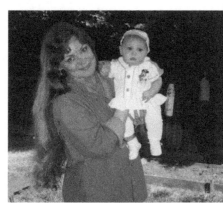
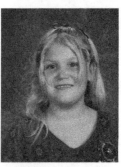
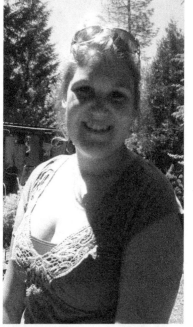
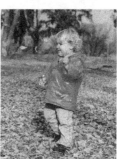
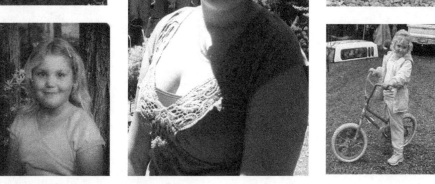
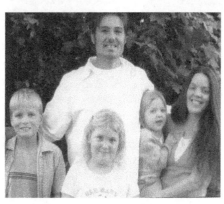
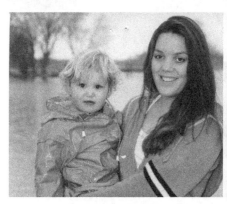

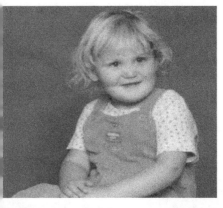
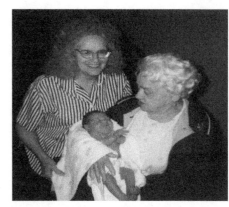
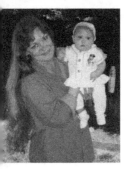
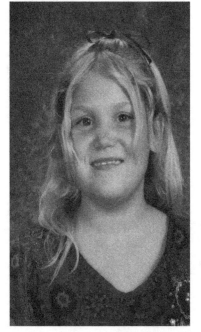
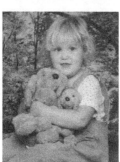
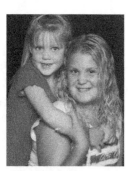
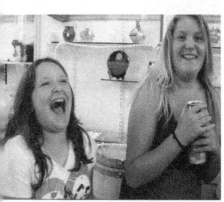
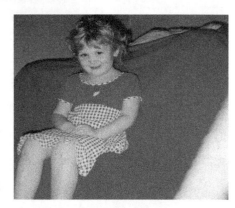

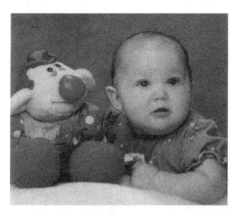
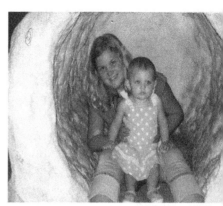
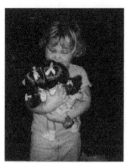
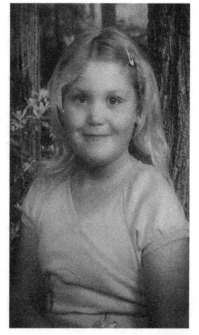
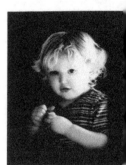
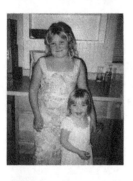
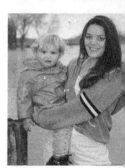
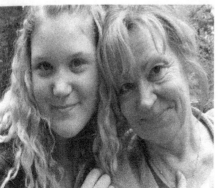
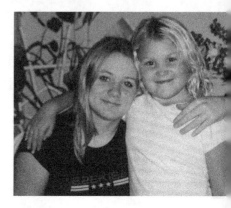

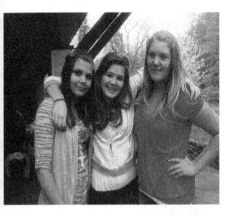
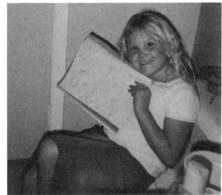
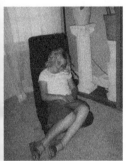
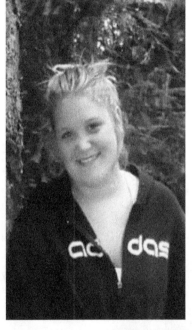
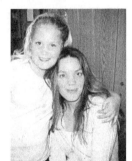
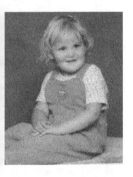
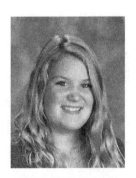
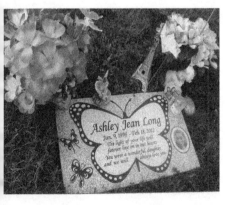

Ashley Jean Long
Jan. 9, 1996 - Feb. 18, 2012

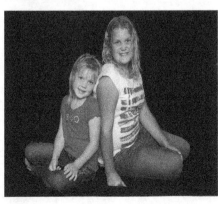

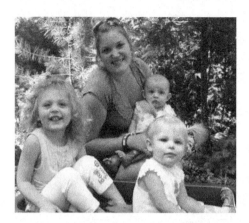
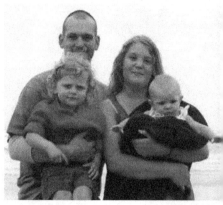
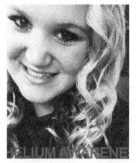
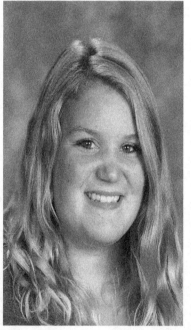
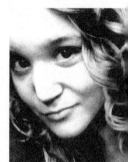
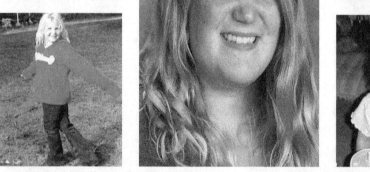
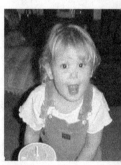
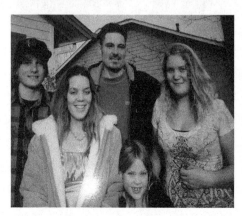
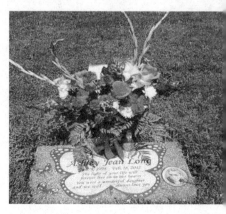

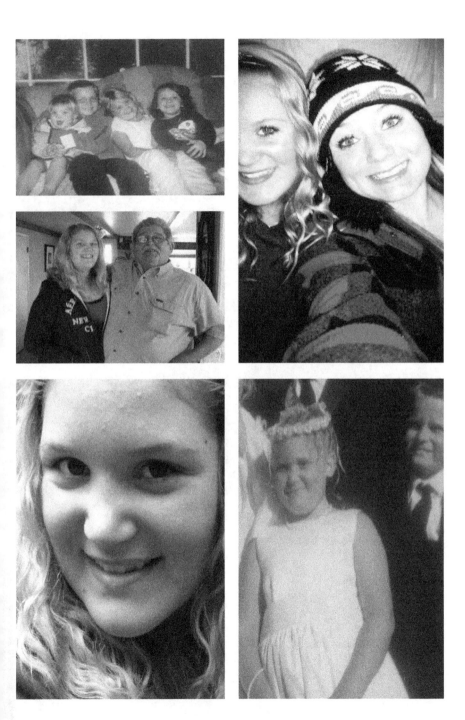

Memorial Day 2017

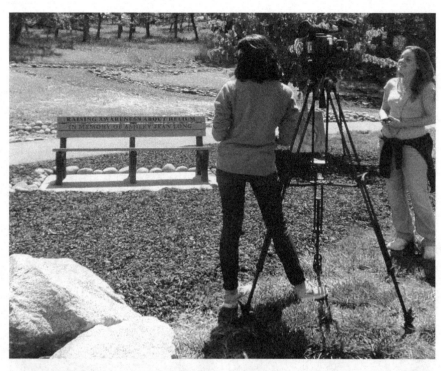

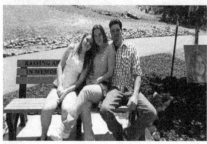

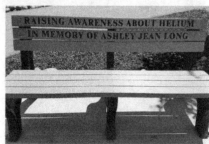

Photos of Jordan McDowell,
another young victim of helium inhalation.

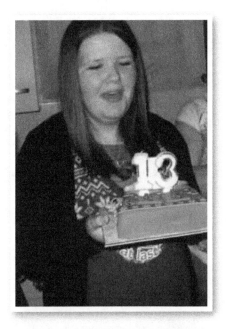

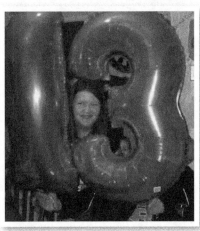

For more tragic stories involving helium and it's hidden dangers, please visit:

Helium Awareness on Facebook

For ways to decorate without using helium, please visit:

Helium Awareness on Pinterest

For information about the danger of helium,
please visit:

Facebook.com/HeliumAwareness

Pinterest.com/loriearp/helium-awareness/

CPSIA information can be obtained
at www.ICGtesting.com
Printed in the USA
LVHW082002100119
603457LV00010B/111/P